Quick And Easy Cookbook: 5 Minute Recipes For Diabetes Management

Diabetes Diet Made Easy With Quick And Easy Recipes

By: Dana Tebow & Mary Lime

ISBN-13: 978-1481859004

Quick And Easy Recipes

Table of Contents

Publishers Notes

Dedication

Chapter 1- The Diabetic Diet

Chapter 2- Breakfast Recipes

Chapter 3- Lunch & Dinner Recipes

Chapter 4- Salads

Chapter 5- Snacks & Desserts

About The Authors

Dana Tebow & Mary Lime

PUBLISHERS NOTES
Disclaimer

This publication is intended to provide helpful and informative material. It is not intended to diagnose, treat, cure, or prevent any health problem or condition, nor is intended to replace the advice of a physician. No action should be taken solely on the contents of this book. Always consult your physician or qualified health-care professional on any matters regarding your health and before adopting any suggestions in this book or drawing inferences from it.

The author and publisher specifically disclaim all responsibility for any liability, loss or risk, personal or otherwise, which is incurred as a consequence, directly or indirectly, from the use or application of any contents of this book.

Any and all product names referenced within this book are the trademarks of their respective owners. None of these owners have sponsored, authorized, endorsed, or approved this book.

Always read all information provided by the manufacturers' product labels before using their products. The author and publisher are not responsible for claims made by manufacturers.

Kindle Edition 2012

Manufactured in the United States of America

Dedication

I want to dedicate this book to my really great team of friends and well wishers who have encouraged me to write about the problem of diabetes and lend my culinary knowledge to creating a great diabetic book.

Chapter 1- The Diabetic Diet

The number of persons with diabetes is increasing and the fact is that a lot of the instances can be prevented with healthy changes to one's lifestyle. There are some situations that can even be reversed. When the right steps are taken to control and prevent diabetes it does not mean that you have to live without eating what you like.

Even though it is essential to eat properly, there is no need to forego sweets entirely or to start eating foods that are bland. With the tips outline below you are still able to enjoy food that you like and get the same pleasure from the meals that you would before without feeling deprived of hungry.

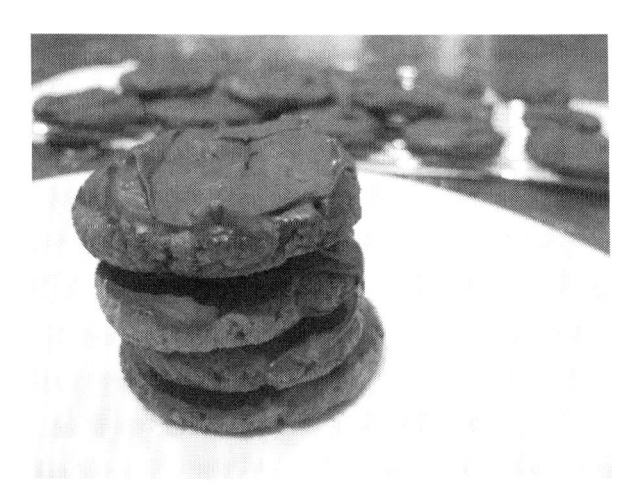

Managing Diabetes

Have you recently been diagnosed with pre-diabetes or diabetes? Have you been warned by the doctor that you are at risk? It can be disheartening to hear that your health is not what you think it is and you may even feel as if you can do nothing about it.

This is a situation that you might be able to relate to. The doctor is advising you that it is essential that you lose weight and make a change to what you are consuming and you are already depressed. The thing is that you have tried to diet beforehand and had no success. The entire process of following the food charts, measuring portion sizes and counting calories seems way too hard.

You Can Get Major Changes from Small Changes

There is some good news whether or not you are trying to control. Or prevent diabetes. With some changes to your lifestyle a big difference can be made. The best thing that you can do in this situation is to lose weight and you do not have to lose all the weight to start benefitting.

The experts state that losing approximately five to ten percent of the weight can lower cholesterol levels as well as blood pressure and blood sugar. It is never too late to start making the changes even if you have already been diagnosed with diabetes. The main point is that you are more in control of your health than you think you are.

All Body Fat Is Different

Being overweight is the biggest risk factor for diabetes but bear in mind that all body fat is different. If the weight is around the abdomen the risk is higher than those that have it around the thighs and hips. The question is why persons with a pear shape are not at as great a risk as those that have an apple shape.

Pear shaped individuals tend to store most of the fat right below the skin while apple shaped individuals store it in the mid region, a lot of it deep in the stomach around the liver and abdominal organs. This kind of fat has a link to diabetes and insulin resistance. A number of studies have indicated that body mass index (BMI) is not as good a predictor of diabetes as the size of the waist.

You stand a greater chance of becoming diabetic if you happen to be:

A male with a waist size that is forty inches or more

A female with a waist size that is thirty five inches or more

To measure the circumference of the waist, put the tape measure just above the hip bone around the abdomen. Ensure that the tape is held tightly but not tight enough to press the skin in. also ensure that it is parallel to the floor. After exhaling and relaxing measure the waist.

What Should Be Known About Diet and Diabetes

Eating properly is essential if you are attempting to control or prevent diabetes, though exercise is extremely important, the food that you eat make the biggest difference when it comes to losing weight. The question is what does that really mean? You might be surprised to learn that the nutritional needs are basically the same as for everyone else. There is no need for a complicated diet or special food.

The diabetes diet is merely sticking to a healthy eating regimen that is moderate in calories, low in fat and high in nutrients. The main difference is that you have to be more careful with some of the food selections- the carbohydrates in particular.

A Few Fallacies about Diet and Diabetes

Quick And Easy Recipes

Fallacy: sugar must not be consumed

Truth: the great news is that you can still eat what you want to as long as the eating plan is sound. Dessert is not off limits either as long as it is healthy or paired with exercise.

Fallacy: the best option is a high protein diet

Truth: research has shown that when too much protein is consumed, particularly animal protein, insulin resistance can be created which plays a major role in diabetes. Fats, carbohydrates and protein are all a part of the healthy diet and the body requires them to work effectively. Balance is the key.

Fallacy: you have to really stop eating those carbs

Truth: Balance is the key. When it comes to carbohydrates serving size is important. The focus has to be placed on whole grain carbs as they are a great source of fiber and as they digest slowly, the levels of blood sugar are more stable.

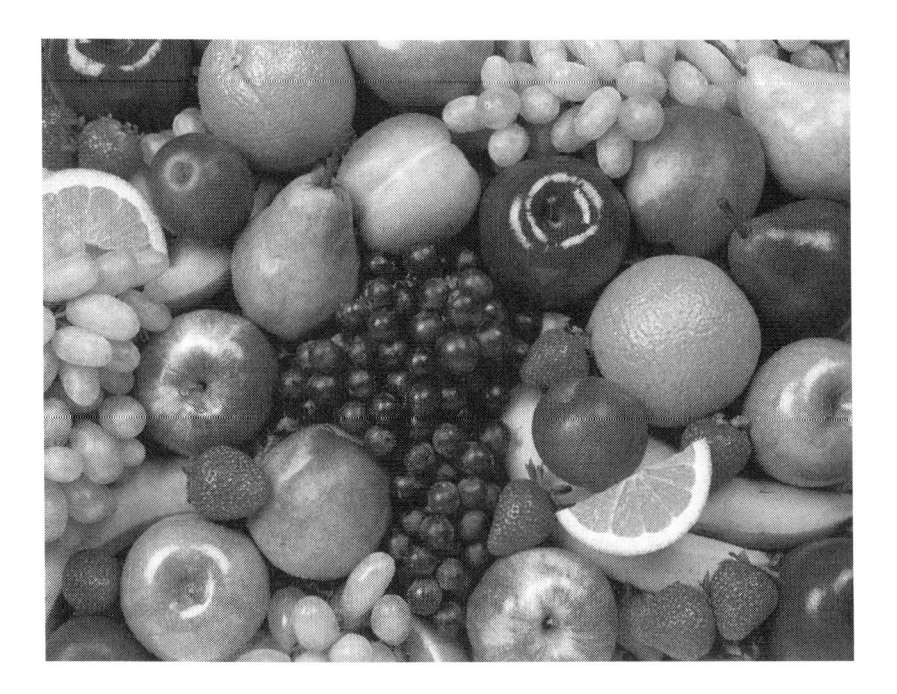

Fallacy: you have to go on a special diet and not eat normally again.

Truth: the principles are the same and it does not matter whether or not you are controlling or preventing diabetes. There really is no added benefit to be gained from the expensive diabetic foods. You can eat with your friends and family as long as you eat in moderation.

Diet and Diabetes Tips

Select Slow Release, High Fiber Carbs

Carbohydrates can affect the levels of blood sugar more so that proteins or fats but they do not have to be eliminated from the diet. One just has to be smart about the carbs that are consumed.

Quick And Easy Recipes

Typically it is prudent to cut down on the consumption of the highly refined carbohydrates like snack foods, candy, soda, rice, pasta and white bread. the focus should be placed on complex carbohydrates that are high in fiber.

These are also known as slow release carbohydrates. These types of carbohydrates help to balance the levels of blood sugar as they get digested more slowly and do not trigger the production of excess insulin. These carbs also keep you full longer and provide energy that lasts.

Be Careful With Sweets

One does not have to eliminate sugar when you are diabetic. If you are diabetic you are still able to enjoy a small bit of your preferred dessert from time to time. Moderation is important.

It may be that you are having a challenge when it comes to reducing the consumption of sweets. The great thing is that you will be able to deal with the cravings and they will eventually become less pronounced and then go away altogether. When the eating habits become healthier the foods that you used to enjoy before may become too sweet or too rich and you will go for the healthier options.

Select Fats Wisely

Fats can either be good or bad. Individuals with diabetes have a greater chance to have heart disease so it is very important to be careful with the fats you consume. A lot of the fats are not healthy while others are extremely beneficial. Portions sizes have to be watched however as all fats are high in calories.

Fats That Are Unhealthy

Trans fats and saturated fats are two of the most harmful fats. Trans fats also known as partially hydrogenated oils are made when hydrogen is added to liquid vegetable oils to get a more solid consistency so things will not spoil as quickly. Saturated fats can be found in eggs, whole dairy products and red meat, all animal products.

Fats That Are Healthy

Unsaturated fats are the best fats and they can be found in fish and plant sources and tend to be liquid at room temperature. The main sources of this fat are avocados, nuts, canola oil and olive oil. The focus should be on omega 3 fatty acids which support heart and brain health and fight inflammation. The best sources include flaxseed, tuna and salmon.

Quick And Easy Recipes

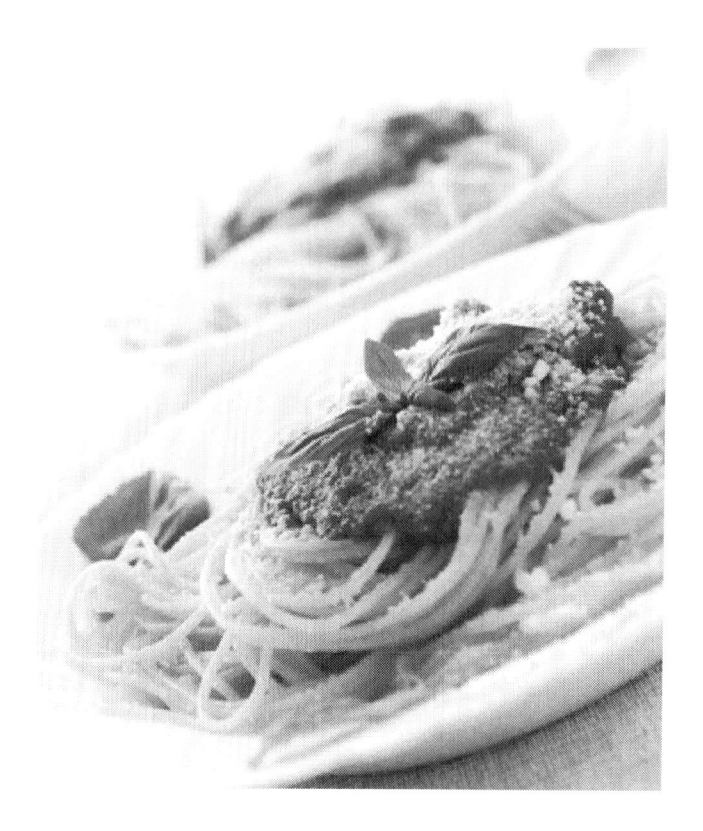

Keep A Food Diary and Eat On A Regular Basis

If you happen to be overweight, you might be happy to learn that you only need to lose approximately seven percent of the body weight to lower the risk of diabetes by fifty percent. There is no need to starve or count calories.

For success with weight loss research indicates that two of the primary actions involve recording what you eat and sticking to a consistent eating schedule.

What Role Does Exercise Play?

As it pertains to reversing, controlling and preventing diabetes exercise cannot be avoided. Exercise can assist you in your efforts for weight loss and is vital to maintaining the loss of weight. Evidence also exists to show that consistent exercise can boost sensitivity to insulin even if no weight is lost.

One does not have to live in the gym or go on some ironman fitness program. The best way to start is by walking every day for approximately thirty minutes each day. Low impact exercises like biking and swimming can be done as well. You will breathe harder and work up a sweat. Even yard work and house work counts.

Chapter 2- Breakfast Recipes
Ginger-Pear Pancakes

1 recipe Apricot-Pear Syrup (recipe below)

½ of a medium pear (cored and finely chop)

2 tablespoons canola oil

¼ cup frozen or refrigerated egg product (or 1 egg)

¾ cup milk (fat-free)

⅛ teaspoon salt

¼ teaspoon ginger (ground)

2 teaspoons baking powder

1 tablespoon packed brown sugar or brown sugar substitute*

½ cup whole wheat flour

½ cup all-purpose flour

In a medium sized bowl, mix salt, ginger, baking powder, brown sugar, whole wheat flour and all purpose flour. In the center of the flour center make a well then set it aside.

Whisk together oil, egg and milk in a small bowl then mix in chopped pear. Put all of the egg mixture in the flour and combine well.

To make each pancake pour a quarter of the batter into a heavy skillet or lightly greased griddle then cook for two to four minutes until the pancakes have a golden color then turn it over and complete cooking.

Dana Tebow & Mary Lime

Serve Apricot Pear Syrup on the pancakes

Tip

Sugar Substitutes: select from sugar twin granulated brown or Sweet'N Low Brown.

Quick And Easy Recipes

Apricot-Pear Syrup

⅛ teaspoon ground ginger

1 tablespoon water

2 tablespoons low sugar apricot preserves

1 tablespoon lemon juice

½ of a cored medium pear (finely chopped)

Combine lemon juice and pear in a small saucepan. Mix in ginger, water and preserves. Heat on low flame until mixture is warm and the preserves are melted stirring frequently.

Dana Tebow & Mary Lime

Sausage with Scrambled Eggs

1 toasted whole grain English muffin (cut in half)

2 tablespoons finely shredded cheddar cheese (reduced-fat)

¼ cup quartered cherry tomatoes

1 ounce sliced cooked turkey sausage

Pinch ground black pepper

2 tablespoons chicken broth (reduced-sodium)

2 eggs

Nonstick cooking spray

Use cooking spray to coat nonstick skillet then preheat on medium fire.

Whisk black pepper, broth, eggs in medium bowl with rotary beater then mix in sliced sausage.

Put the mixture into the skillet then let cook until mixtures starts to set around the edges and on the bottom.

Wait a large spoon or spatula lift then fold to allow the rest of mixture to flow underneath. Continue to cook on medium flame until almost complete then add cheese and tomatoes. Cook for another minute.

Serve on toasted English muffin halves.

Quick And Easy Recipes

Blueberry Compote with Cornmeal Waffles

1 recipe Blueberry Compote (see below)

2 egg whites

½ teaspoon vanilla

2 egg yolks

3 tablespoons canola oil

½ cup milk (fat-free)

1 cup buttermilk

¼ teaspoon salt

1 teaspoon baking powder

*2 tablespoons packed brown sugar**

½ cup cornmeal

¾ cup flour

Mix salt, baking powder, brown sugar, cornmeal and flour in a large bowl.

Mix vanilla, egg yolks, oil, milk and buttermilk in a medium bowl whisking to combine properly then add to flour and combine.

Use an electric mixture to beat egg whites in a large bowl until soft peaks are formed, then fold the egg whites into batter gently.

Tips

Dana Tebow & Mary Lime

If you are utilizing a waffle iron that is six inches round use half cup of batter for each waffle and serve three quarters per serving.

*Sugar Substitutes: select from sugar twin granulated brown and Sweet'N Low Brown and use directions on package to use equivalent amounts.

Quick And Easy Recipes

Blueberry Compote

⅛ teaspoon cinnamon (ground)

½ teaspoon lemon peel (finely shredded)

2 cups blueberries (fresh)

1 tablespoon lemon juice

1 cup apple juice

Bring lemon juice and apple juice to a boil in a medium saucepan then lower heat. Let simmer uncovered for eight to ten minutes or until it is reduced. Mix in cinnamon, lemon peel and fresh blue berries. Allow to boil again and then lower heat.

Dana Tebow & Mary Lime

Breakfast Shake

1 cup non fat yogurt or fat free milk

½ cup fruit

1 tsp. wheat germ

1 tsp. nut butter or nuts

Blend wheat germ with fruit and non fat yogurt or fat free milk then add nut butter or nuts and ice.

Quick And Easy Recipes

Muffin and Berries

Small bran muffin

Fresh berries

Fresh yogurt

Split bran muffin and after placing it on plate then top berries and yogurt.

Chutney and Bagel

On a small bagel spread mango chutney then add cottage cheese and sprinkle it with cinnamon.

Cheese and Baked Potato

½ medium potato

Salsa

Low fat cheddar cheese

Place a spoonful of salsa and low fat cheese on top half of medium potato. Heat in microwave until cheese melts.

Dana Tebow & Mary Lime

Microwave Poached Eggs

Ingredients:

Pepper and salt

⅓ cup water

⅛ teaspoon white vinegar

1 large egg

Directions:

In six ounce custard cup add white vinegar and water.

Use toothpick to pierce egg yolk after breaking egg into cup then use plastic wrap to loosely cover dish.

Put in microwave and cook for a minute.

Depending on the microwave you have it may require more or less time.

When done take egg out immediately then serve with pepper and salt to taste.

Quick And Easy Recipes

Pumpkin Shake

Ingredients:

1 teaspoon vanilla

⅛ teaspoon cinnamon

8 teaspoons sugar ("or" substitute sweetener)

1 ½ cups cold skim milk

4 ounces canned pumpkin (chilled)

Directions:

Mix all ingredients in a blender.

Chapter 3 - Lunch & Dinner Recipes

Black Bean and Beef Wraps

1½ cups shredded Monterey jack cheese or cheddar (4 to 6 ounces)

1½ cups lettuce (shredded)

6 eight inch whole wheat flour tortillas

¼ teaspoon black pepper

¼ teaspoon salt

1 large chopped tomato

1 15 ounce can rinsed and drained black beans

½ teaspoon ground coriander

1 teaspoon chili powder

1½ teaspoons cumin (ground)

1 cup onion (chopped)

8 ounces lean ground beef

2 cloves minced garlic

Salsa (optional)

Cook garlic, onion and ground beef in a large skillet until meat is brown (5 minutes) then drain the fat off.

Quick And Easy Recipes

Mix in coriander, chili powder and cumin then cook fir another minute. Mix in black pepper, salt, tomato and black beans then cover and cook for another five minutes stirring frequently.

When serving place beef mixture in the center of the tortillas then sprinkle with cheese and lettuce. Serve with salsa if desired.

Dana Tebow & Mary Lime

Five Minute Quesadillas

Ingredients

1 tsp fresh green onion (chopped)

1 tbsp finely chopped red bell peppers

1 slice Muenster Cheese (other cheese can be used)

1 low carb tortilla (10 inch)

Directions

Top tortilla with vegetables and cheese then fold in half and place on microwaveable plate.

Microwave until cheese melts (fifteen to twenty seconds) then fold in half

Quick And Easy Recipes

Applesauce Quesadillas

Ingredients

1 pinch ground cinnamon

1 tbsp melted margarine, (trans fat free)

⅔ cup cheddar cheese (shredded)

⅔ cup applesauce (unsweetened)

4 low carb tortillas (10 inch)

Directions

Preheat oven to four hundred degrees Fahrenheit then arrange the tortillas on a baking sheet. Over tortillas spoon the applesauce then sprinkle with cinnamon and cheese if you want.

Put the other two tortillas on top and brush with margarine then sprinkle on cinnamon.

Bake tortillas until golden then slice into triangle and serve.

Dana Tebow & Mary Lime

Pineapple Sandwich and Barbecue Chicken

4 hamburger Buns (reduced calorie)

4 piece pineapple slices (canned)

⅓ cup hickory flavored barbeque Sauce

4 fresh red Onion rings

4 chicken breasts (boneless and skinless)

1 cooking spray

Turn the grill on then use cooking spray to spray rack

Use barbeque sauce to coat onion and chicken. Cover and grill pineapple, onion and chicken for five minutes then turn over and grill foe another five minutes.

On bottom of bun put slice put chicken breast then top with pineapple and onion then put on top of bun.

Quick And Easy Recipes

Noodle Beefsteak Tomato Caprese

6 oz Noodles

1 oz crushed fire roasted tomatoes (canned)

⅛ tsp black pepper

⅛ tsp salt

2 tbsp olive oil

3 oz red onion

1 medium tomato

1½ oz chopped fresh basil

2 oz cubed mozzarella (part skim shredded)

Slice the red onion and tomato (put tomato juice aside) and place on plate

Put sliced mozzarella on top and sprinkle with basil (1 ounce)

Toss tomato juice, cubed mozzarella, and remainder of basil, roasted tomatoes and Noodles in a small bowl

Place Noodles beside cheese onion and stacked tomato then add a pinch of pepper and salt then serve.

Dana Tebow & Mary Lime

Banana Berry Shake

4 ice cubes

¼ cup wheat germ

1 cup fresh strawberries (halved)

1 cup milk (fat free)

1 cup cranberry Juice (unsweetened)

1 large banana (cut in chunks)

Place all ingredients in blender and process until consistency is smooth

Other Information

Variation:

Instead of bananas and strawberries use 2 cups cubed cantaloupe

Use 1 cup orange juice instead of cranberry juice

Quick And Easy Recipes

Boiled Edamame

1 tsp sea salt or salt (to taste)

2 lb frozen Soybeans, edamame (with pod)

1 tsp salt

Mix salt and three quarts of water in a big pot and let come to a boil. Add the soybean and cook until soybeans are tender (five minutes) then strain and season with salt. Serve chilled or warm.

Other Information

Be careful not to undercook or overcook soybeans

Broiled Crab Cakes

Cooking spray

1 pinch Tabasco sauce

1 egg

1 ½ oz minced yellow onion

2 tbsp Dijon mustard

2 tbsp mayonnaise

1 ½ lb raw blue Crab (shells and cartilage removed)

Preheat the broiler then use cooking spray to lightly coat broiler pan

Mix all ingredients in a bowl

Make 6 round cakes from mixture then place in broiler pan

Place pan under broiler approximately six inches from the heat then cook on each side for three minutes until they are browned lightly.

Quick And Easy Recipes

Special California Wrap

1 tbsp fat free ranch Salad Dressing

1 fresh sprig of arugula or watercress

1 tsp lime juice (fresh)

1 piece sliced fresh medium California avocado (⅛ of medium)

1 small sliced tomato

1 piece honey baked ham lunchmeat

1 piece 95% fat free slice turkey lunchmeat (oven roasted white meat)

1 green lettuce leaf

On plate fan out the lettuce then top with tomato, ham and turkey

Mix lime juice and avocado in small bowl then spoon it onto the tomato

Top with arugula or watercress and the dressing then roll it and secure it using a wooden toothpick.

Dana Tebow & Mary Lime

Veggie and Cheese Sandwiches

1 small tomato (cut into 4 slices)

2 oz fresh lettuce leaves or spinach leaves

2 tbsp horseradish mustard

8 piece sliced whole grain bread

¼ cup plain yogurt (low fat)

½ tsp finely snipped fresh chives

¼ cup fresh chopped green sweet pepper or celery

¼ cup carrots (shredded)

1 ½ cup 1% fat Cottage Cheese (drained)

Mix chives, green pepper, celery, carrot and cottage cheese in a medium bowl then mix in yogurt.

On whole grain bread spread horseradish evenly then put spinach over the slices of bread. Put the mixture of cottage cheese over the spinach then put slice of tomato on top and cover with remaining slices of bread.

Quick And Easy Recipes

Cheesy Pita

1 cup shredded fat free cheddar cheese

¼ tsp hot red pepper flakes (optional)

¼ cup fresh green onion (chopped)

1 finely chopped fresh plum tomato

2 oz finely chopped small green bell peppers

2 frozen Vegetarian Meat (light sausage) - slice into pieces ¼ inch thick

2 large pitas (whole wheat)

Preheat the oven to four hundred and seventy five degrees

Slice each pita in half carefully then place them on baking sheet.

On top place the patties then the bell pepper and tomato then green onion and red pepper flakes and the cheese then baked until the cheese is melted (five minutes)

Cheesy Pizza with Spinach

½ cup crumbled Feta Cheese

½ cup shredded mozzarella (part skim)

10 oz thin Pizza Crust (ready to heat)

½ cup chopped Artichoke hearts (canned, marinated rinsed and drained)

8 oz fresh baby spinach (in a microwavable bag)

Preheat the broiler

Place spinach in microwave and cook based on direction on the package then coarsely chop spinach and put in a medium sized bowl then stir in the artichokes.

On a baking sheet place the pizza crust, place in broiler approximately five inches from source of heat for thirty to sixty seconds per side (until golden).

Carefully take the pan out and leave the broiler on then spread mixture over crust evenly leaving one inch on edge free. Use both cheese to top evenly then broil until the feta is partially melted and mozzarella is completely melted (fifty to seventy seconds) then cut in wedges and serve.

Quick And Easy Recipes

Chicken Salad with Blue Cheese and Dates

1 ½ oz crumbled blue Cheese

¼ tsp salt

3 tbsp sugar

¼ cup balsamic vinegar

½ cup dates (chopped)

9 oz cooked diced chicken breast

½ cup thinly sliced red onion

8 cup salad greens

1 ½ oz oriental flavor ramen noodle Soup (dry, serving)

1 oz chopped walnuts (or pecans)

Over medium high heat, heat nonstick skillet then add noodle soup mix and nuts and cook for two to three minutes and remove from heat and place aside.

Divide greens, dates, chicken and onions evenly divided on 4 plates

To make dressing pour salt, sugar and vinegar in a jar then cover and shake to mix

Drizzle each plate with dressing then sprinkle with blue cheese.

Dana Tebow & Mary Lime

Crab Pitas

3 oz softened cream cheese (low fat)

½ lb crabmeat (imitation)

2 fresh chopped green onions

12 small whole wheat pitas (halved)

Put green onions imitation crabmeat and cream cheese in food processor bowl then process until consistency is smooth

On each half of pita spoon 1 table spoon carb mix and serve

Quick And Easy Recipes

Marinara with Cottage Cheese

¼ cup marinara sauce (low sodium)

2 ½ tbsp shredded Mozzarella Cheese (reduced fat)

½ cup cottage cheese (fat free)

Mix mozzarella cheese, cottage cheese and marinara sauce in a small microwavable bowl

Microwave until mixture is hot and mozzarella is melted, (one to two minutes on medium power) then serve at once

Dana Tebow & Mary Lime

Cucumber Dunkers with Fast Guacamole

2 medium avocados

½ cup salsa

¼ fl oz hot pepper sauce (optional)

1 medium seeded and sliced cucumber (slice in rounds ⅛ inch thick)

1 pinch pepper and salt (to taste)

Cut the avocados in half then remove the pits and discard them. In a medium bowl scoop the flesh and the use a fork to mash.

Add hot pepper sauce and salsa to mashed avocado and combine well

Put guacamole in a serving bowl and place cucumber chips around it.

CHAPTER 4- SALADS
Spinach Chorizo Salad

2 tbsp sherry vinegar

5 oz thinly sliced chorizo sausage

6 tbsp olive oil (extra virgin)

8 oz baby spinach (fresh)

Start by getting rid of the tough stalks that the spinach has

Next in a large frying pan add oil then put in the sausage and cook it for three minutes. When it is finished the slices ought to start to change color and shrivel a bit.

Place the spinach leaves in the pan then take if off the heat and toss the spinach until it begins to wilt.

Add a little seasoning and sherry vinegar then toss to combine and serve while it is still warm

Spinach Salad and Roasted Red Peppers

1 tablespoon reduced-fat feta cheese (crumbled)

2 tablespoons toasted whole pecans and almonds

3 tablespoons drained and sliced roasted red sweet peppers (jarred)

2 cups fresh baby spinach (packaged)

⅛ teaspoon black pepper

1 clove minced garlic

1 teaspoon sugar or sugar substitute* equivalent to 1 teaspoon sugar

1 teaspoon olive oil

2 tablespoons cider vinegar

1 slice turkey bacon

To make dressing:

Cook bacon in a medium skillet then take it out of the skillet and let cool slightly then chop and set aside. Use the same skillet and whisk black pepper, garlic, sugar, oil and vinegar. Let boil then turn heat down and stir frequently for another minute.

Mix feta cheese, almonds, roasted peppers, spinach and chopped bacon in a medium bowl then drizzle with warm dressing and toss to coat then serve.

Quick And Easy Recipes

Salad of Superfoods

½ teaspoon freshly ground black pepper

1 ounce crumbled semisoft goat cheese

¼ cup coarsely chopped and toasted walnuts

½ cup fresh blueberries

2 cups hulled and sliced fresh strawberries

2 cups cooked chicken breast (chopped)

4 cups fresh baby spinach leaves (packaged)

¼ teaspoon salt

1 tablespoon canola oil

2 tablespoons honey

2 tablespoons fresh mint (snipped)

⅓ cup raspberry vinegar

To make vinaigrette:

In a jar with a screw on top mix salt, oil, honey, mint and vinegar then cover and shake to mix.

Toss goat cheese, walnuts, blueberries, strawberries, chicken and spinach in a large bowl then place salad in plates. Drizzle with vinaigrette and sprinkle with pepper.

Dana Tebow & Mary Lime

Chicken Salad

2 tablespoons reduced-fat feta cheese (crumbled)

2 tablespoons pitted and quartered kalamata olives

1 15 ounce can rinsed and drained chickpeas (garbanzo beans)

2 plum tomatoes (cut in wedges)

2 cups cooked chicken breast (cut-up)

5 cups romaine lettuce (shredded)

¼ teaspoon ground black pepper

1 tablespoon honey

2 tablespoons olive oil

2 tablespoons fresh basil (snipped)

2 tablespoons fresh mint (snipped)

⅓ cup lemon juice

Whole kalamata olives (optional)

To make dressing:

In a jar with a screw top put pepper, honey, oil, basil, mint and lemon juice then cover and shake well to mix.

On a large platter arrange the lettuce then top with chicken, cheese, tomatoes, beans and quartered olives (if desired). Drizzle with dressing then garnish with whole olives

Quick And Easy Recipes

Basil Vinaigrette on a Scallop Salad

2 tablespoons Parmesan cheese- finely shredded (optional)

½ of a medium English cucumber (chopped)

1 cup frozen whole kernel corn (thaw) or fresh corn kernels

1 medium seeded and chopped red sweet pepper

3 plum seeded and chopped tomatoes

1 pound frozen or fresh sea scallops

6 cups torn mixed salad greens

Nonstick cooking spray

½ teaspoon ground black pepper

2 teaspoons mustard (Dijon-style)

2 tablespoons olive oil

2 tablespoons lemon juice

3 tablespoons balsamic vinegar

¼ cup fresh basil (snipped)

If scallops are frozen let them thaw then rinse them and use paper towels to pat dry.

To make vinaigrette in a jar with screw top mix ¼ teaspoon black pepper, mustard, oil, lemon juice, vinegar and basil. Cover and shake then set aside.

Use rest of black pepper to sprinkle scallops. Use cooking spray to coat large nonstick skillet then preheat. Cook scallops until they are opaque (two to four minutes turning them halfway through the cooking process.

In the meantime serve salad on four plates. Combine cucumber, corn, sweet pepper and tomatoes in a large bowl then serve on plates as well then serve scallops and use remaining vinaigrette to brush them. Sprinkle with Parmesan cheese if desired.

Quick And Easy Recipes

Broccoli & Turkey with Grapes

⅛ teaspoon black pepper (coarsely ground)

¼ cup toasted slivered or sliced sunflower kernels or slivered almonds

1 cup carrot (coarsely shredded)

1½ cups halved red grapes (seedless)

1 pound cooked shredded turkey breast

1 12 ounce package shredded broccoli (broccoli slaw mix)

⅛ teaspoon salt

2 teaspoons sugar substitute* or sugar

2 tablespoons olive oil

⅓ cup white balsamic vinegar

To make vinaigrette:

Mix salt, sugar, oil and vinegar in a jar with a screw top.

In a big bowl mix carrot, grapes, turkey and shredded broccoli then put on dressing and toss to coat. Cover and place in refrigerator to chill for twenty four hours or serve immediately. Before serving, add almonds.

*Sugar Substitutes:

Select between Sweet 'N Low, Equal or Splenda Granular. Follow instructions on package to use correct amount.

Chapter 5 - Snacks & Desserts

Simple Cucumber Cups

1 sprig dill (fresh -split into twelve sections)

¼ cup hummus

¼ cup reduced fat sour cream

1 tablespoon mustard (horseradish)

1 peeled English cucumber (seedless)

½ cup peas*

* Thawed frozen peas or canned peas with no salt added can be used

Cut cucumber into two inch rounds (approximately twelve pieces) then scoop the inner flesh out taking care not to scoop through the bottom. Places slice to drain on cotton or paper towels.

Use immersion blender or regular blender to puree sour cream, mustard and peas or simply use a fork to mash ingredients.

Place two teaspoons of hummus in each cucumber cup then fill with pea mixture and use sprig of dill to garnish.

Quick And Easy Recipes

Blueberry Peach Parfaits

¼ teaspoon ground cinnamon

½ cup blueberries (fresh)

1 pitted and cut up ripe peach

1 cup multigrain clusters cereal (lightly sweetened)

1 6 ounce carton fat free blueberry, peach or vanilla yogurt

In two bowls or dessert glasses share the yogurt then use half of cereal to top it. Add the cinnamon, half the blueberries and half the peaches in each. Repeat the process until bowls or glasses are full.

Dana Tebow & Mary Lime

Apricot Yogurt

2 tsp sugar substitute (sweetener)

8 oz non fat sugar free mango apricot yogurt

¼ cup low sugar apricot preserves

In small bowl whisk apricot spread

Add sugar substitute and yogurt

Whisk to blend then serve in dessert bowls.

Quick And Easy Recipes

Raspberry, Banana and Cottage Cheese Split

½ cup fresh raspberries

1 medium peeled and sectioned orange

½ cup non fat cottage cheese

1 fresh medium banana

In each bowl place half a banana then top with quarter cup cottage cheese. Place oranges around the cheese

Place raspberries in blender and blend until consistency is smooth then pour it over the bananas then serve.

Dana Tebow & Mary Lime

Banana Snack

1 tbsp reduced sodium peanut butter

1 fresh medium banana

After cutting the banana in half slice it down the middle then put peanut butter between half of banana. Use saran wrap to wrap it then put it in freezer for two hours.

Quick And Easy Recipes

Barbeque Popcorn

1 cooking spray (butter flavored)

8 cup air popped popcorn

½ tsp garlic powder

½ tsp ground cumin

1 tsp onion powder

1 tsp hickory smoked salt

1 tbsp paprika

Mix garlic powder, cumin, onion powder, hickory smoked salt and paprika in a bowl.

Place popcorn on large baking sheet with rim then spray with nonstick butter

Sprinkle spice mix on popcorn then toss to coat and serve.

Dana Tebow & Mary Lime

Happy Snack Mix

½ cup milk chocolate morsels baking chips

½ cup raisins (seedless)

1 cup honey roasted peanuts

2 cup cheerios cereal

16 oz Crackers (squares, honey, graham) - mini grahams that are bear-shaped

In a re-sealable bag or large bowl mix all the ingredients. Store in an airtight container

Quick And Easy Recipes

Mix of Berries

½ medium squeezed lemons

1 medium squeezed orange

½ cup granulated Splenda

1 lb fresh blueberries

1 lb fresh sliced strawberries (no stem)

Mix blueberries and strawberries in a large bowl

Mix lemon juice, orange juice and confectioners' sugar in small bowl and stir to dissolve sugar

Pour the juice on the fruit and toss gently then serve

Tip

To reduce use of sugar use granulated sugar substitute or use under half cup of sugar.

Dana Tebow & Mary Lime

Nutty & Berry Snack Mix

1¼ cup whole salted cashew nuts

6 oz dried cranberries

7 2/5 oz cheddar cheese crackers

Mix cashews, cranberries and crackers then store in airtight container.

Tip

Use any other nuts and dried fruit to make this quick snack

Quick And Easy Recipes

Quick Popcorn

⅛ Tsp salt

1 butter spray

¼ cup yellow popcorn (not popped)

Put kernels in brown paper bag seal and place in microwave and pop

Take bag out of microwave and spray popcorn with spray then seal and shake, repeat two times then add salt.

Dana Tebow & Mary Lime

Celery Snack

1 pinch paprika

8 oz crushed pineapple in juice (drain)

8 oz cream cheese (low fat)

15 small fresh celery stalks

Trim the celery stalks then wash and dry

Mix pineapple and cream cheese then spoon mix into celery and use a knife to level.

Lightly sprinkle with paprika then cover and let chill

Serve celery after cutting into two inch pieces

Quick And Easy Recipes

Apple & Cheese Crunch

¼ sliced medium apples

½ oz Splenda with sugar free apricot preserves

2 tbsp creamy natural peanut butter

1 rice cake (multigrain and brown rice)

½ oz sharp cheddar cheese

Spread peanut butter on rice cake or multigrain

Mix chopped apple and preserves then spoon onto peanut butter.

Sprinkle on cheese and serve

Dana Tebow & Mary Lime

Caramelized Strawberries and Cantaloupe

½ a cantaloup

1 tbsp confectioners' sugar (have extra for dusting)

1 cup fresh strawberries

Start by preheating broiler of high setting.

Hull strawberries then cut them in half and in an ovenproof dish or on a baking sheet arrange fruit cut side up in a single layer. Use 1 tablespoon powdered sugar to dust.

Place strawberries in broiler until they start turning golden brown and sugar starts to bubble (*four to five minutes*). While strawberries are in broiler use spoon to get seeds out of melon then use a sharp knife to remove skin.

Cut flesh of melon into wedges then arrange on serving plate and place strawberries on top. Use extra sugar to dust and serve at once.

Quick And Easy Recipes

Cereal Treats

5 cups crispy rice cereal

10 ½ oz marshmallows (miniature)

¼ cup unsalted butter

1 cooking spray

Use cooking or butter spray to crease 9 x 13 pan.

Mix marshmallows and butter in microwave safe bowl then microwave on high setting for one or two minutes. Stir every thirty seconds or so until it is smooth. Remove it from the oven and add cereal.

Add mixture to greased pan pressing it in using the back of a spoon that is buttered. Allow it to cool then cut into squares and serve.

Dana Tebow & Mary Lime

Apples and Cheddar Cheese

2 oz sharp cheddar cheese (reduced fat)

1 tbsp lemon juice (fresh)

2 apples (small)

Cut apple into thin slices after coring it

Serve onto two plates and use lemon juice to sprinkle it

Slice the cheese and serve over the slices.

Quick And Easy Recipes

Ginger & Tropical Fruits

2 tsp grated fresh ginger root

⅓ Cup orange juice

1 small banana (cut into piece ¼ inch thick

2 cup diced pineapple (fresh)

1 peeled fresh mango (remove the seeds and cut mango into cubes)

In a bowl mix all the ingredients then serve immediately

Other Information

Different fruits can be used.

Dana Tebow & Mary Lime

Tangy Fruit Salad

2 fl oz aromatic bitters

½ cup fresh seedless grapes (halved)

2 peeled and thinly sliced navel oranges

Mix bitters and grapes in mixing bowl

On a platter arrange the orange slices then spoon grape mix over it

Cover it and place in refrigerator until it is time to be served

Other Information

Use blood oranges to add interesting taste and color to the recipe.

Quick And Easy Recipes

Simple Fruit Dip

1 cup bran flakes cereal

8 oz thawed light whipped topping

6 cups sliced frozen fruit (pineapple, peach and strawberry) - any fresh fruit can be used

In bowl dip the fruit into the whipped topping to coat then sprinkle with cereal and serve immediately.

Dana Tebow & Mary Lime

Blueberries with Ginger Ale

3 cup blueberries (fresh)

¼ cup orange juice

¼ cup diet ginger ale soda

Put all the blueberries in a bowl

Mix ginger ale and orange juice and spoon this mix over the blueberries then serve.

Other Information

Use other fruits like melon, blackberries, raspberries and strawberries.

Quick And Easy Recipes

ABOUT THE AUTHORS

Dana Tebow is no stranger to diets so writing a book that is specific to diabetes is nothing strange for her. She saw the need to write this book as she noticed the number of persons in her family and community that were being diagnosed with various forms of diabetes. This was of great concern to her as she was familiar with losing loved ones due to their health issues.

She made the decision to get a cook book out that would help everyone not just diabetics to eat much healthier and reduce the chances of early mortality. The great thing is that she is aware that one of the major problems that people have is the lack of time to prepare a wholesome meal as they are always on the go. She solved that by putting together some recipes that are quick to prepare.

The meals are also very tasty. The only thing missing from them is the unnecessary sugars, carbohydrates and fats that can make the problem worse. Dana goes a step further by providing some quick tips as well on the disease. Through her books Dana's aim is to educate and make individuals healthy one person at a time.

Mary Lime is all too familiar with the process of careful selection of what she eats as she is gluten intolerant like other members in her household. As such the transition had to be made by all to a diet free from gluten to keep the possibility of cross contamination at zero.

She has done her research over the years and had put together a rough manual as a guide for herself and her family on things to do and what foods to purchase etc when her husband suggested that she put it in print for others that share the same fate.

After careful consideration she chose to do so as she was more than fully aware of the challenges an individual in her situation might face especially when it came down to shopping for foodstuff every week. Her books isn't overwhelming by any means and provides a wealth of information that any celiac/gluten intolerant individual would find extremely useful.

The transition is not as hard as many may feel as the menu options are just as filling and may even be tastier in some instances than what they used to consume beforehand. In the long run Mary has presented a much healthier and safer way to eat.

Printed in Great Britain
by Amazon